Starting the Fire:

A Beginners Guide on Health and Fitness

By: Kane Eldrick

Disclaimer:

The information contained in this book is for general information purposes only. You should not rely on this information as a substitute for, nor does it replace, professional medical advice, diagnosis, or treatment. The author and publisher assume no responsibility for errors or omissions in the contents of this book. In no event shall the author or publisher be liable for any special, direct, indirect, consequential, or incidental damages or any damages whatsoever, whether in an action of contract, negligence or other tort, arising out of or in connection with the contents of this book.

Contents

——

Introduction

———

This book is intended to introduce core aspects of health and fitness to beginners so that by the time they have finished reading, they will have enough tools to begin improving their health and well-being through diet and exercise. The exercises listed do not require expensive equipment in order to perform and will help the aspirant lay a solid ground work to propel them into more advanced levels of fitness if they so desire. I do not, however, list out specific meal plans and instead provide a perspective that allows one to experiment with their current diet, transforming it into something to be proud of. As this is a guide for beginners, the nutritional information and exercises are short and simplified.

This book is not intended to be your sole resource on health and fitness and I strongly encourage you to do your own research as it is very important to have the capacity to learn on your own. Accompanying research while working through this book will both reinforce knowledge and help keep motivation levels high. I recommend approaching all new information with healthy skepticism but keep in mind that we must be willing to investigate or else it's just doubt and disbelief. I have striven to keep the book short and straight to the point as to avoid intimidating the reader and have placed a bullet point summary at the end of each section to make things easier.

Habits

———

The power of habit is your number one tool to achieve greater health, fitness and anything else for that matter. While passion can often be a strong motivator at first, once it starts to wane we find ourselves with a half developed skill and no desire to continue; this is where the power to make and break habits comes into play. There is much talk of the supposed 21 days to form a new habit but we are all different, as long as it sticks, that's what counts!

So we have vague goal of starting something new and sticking with it for around 3 weeks or so, what else is there to forming habits? Well, for one thing, the new habit has to be realistic or else we will quickly lose motivation. There are all these pressures to jump right into a new diet, immediately start working out 5 days a week and I'd say that most people fail to make these into habits. What I am suggesting here is to start absolutely as small as you would like, we want the new behavior to take root so once it does, it will have its own momentum to help you keep going.

There is, however, a catch to starting really small when it comes to things like strength training and stretching and that is that we must exercise each area of our body in turn to avoid injury. Say you fancy yourself a manly man and you decide to work out by just doing bench presses and bicep curls (why this is manly is beyond me). Over time, you will see your gains diminish and as your biceps and chest continue to tighten and get stronger, your upper back and shoulders will slowly lose their power of support and your strength will have become impractical.

So the habit we want to make can be as small as we want as long as it won't knock us out of balance as to avoid injuring ourselves, that's never fun. Imbalance can occur in an ill-advised diet as well. For example, I have a friend who became determined to improve their health through a vegan diet but things didn't go as well as they had hoped and they acquired a B vitamin deficiency. My friend went in without doing much research and had improvised green smoothies and ate salads and nuts for a few weeks and even with the best of intentions, he achieved mixed results.

When it comes time to choose what exercises and stretches you wish to undertake it's very important that you find balance in the regimen. I include stretching because just as pairs of muscles must be trained evenly so too will it be necessary to stretch with strength training as it is another example of the yin and yang of physical fitness. The act of moving requires both muscles and tendons so if one was to neglect stretching the tendons in favor of muscular strength then they will eventually become imbalanced and lead to some sort of injury not to mention slow down progress.

We are given our greatest examples of the power of consistency through our very own bad habits and addictions. We all have bad habits and while they seem to be our weaknesses, it is in them that we can find our greatest strengths. Our bad habits and addictions are our ways of coping with the various voids in our life. Take drug addiction (to which I include caffeine, alcohol and even sugar), you take your chemical of choice and for a time, you feel more like how you think you should... but for a price. The price we pay for our addictions is tolerance and dependence which moves us further away from good health. We can even find addiction in our relationships. Say you are a very people pleasing kind of individual, always trying to avoid hurting people's feelings but you find yourself dating really strong independent people who just seem to hurt you repeatedly without batting an eye. This type of relationship is like an addiction, the girl is overly merciful and seeks strength through the men that she dates and those men are power oriented people with very little mercy and thus date merciful women. The answer to overcoming bad habits and addictions is to cultivate the attribute that the addiction fulfills so that we don't feel like we need it anymore.

-Summary-

- Start as small as you want with your new habits as long as you're sure it won't knock you out of balance.
- Strength training and stretching are both necessary to become stronger.

- Balance, Balance, Balance
- Addictions fill voids in our life, cultivate the attribute that the addiction fulfills to overcome the addiction

Motivation

——

Through the power of habit we have our ball rolling with decent momentum to our goal, but what should we do on those days where it seems we have every excuse to avoid holding true? What about those days where we go through the motions with minimal effort? How do we keep pushing through when sickness strikes and all we want to do is sit and watch TV with a bunch of comfort food. What we need to do is learn to tap into that part of ourselves that craves exercise and good health and we have many tools available to us to help us get there.

Immersion is an extremely powerful way to accelerate our progress but it does have some draw backs as it will suck energy away from other areas of your life. To become immersed in a goal you need to spend a lot of time with the subject matter of your goal. I'm talking about spending 3+ hours every single day reading, watching videos, journaling, making charts and talking about the intricacies of your goals. This is like forcing passion all the time and it can actually be unhealthy though it will certainly speed up results. If you aren't looking to become obsessed then this probably isn't for you.

Keeping a record of your diet and/or exercise is a fantastic way to increase your morale. For your diet just write down what and how much you eat everyday grouped into meals and snacks. As for your workouts, log each type of exercise with sets, reps and time if applicable. Recording our experiences helps us to see our progress which is very motivating and adds more effort towards our goals which is always good. While I recommend writing it all out yourself, you can very easily find health and fitness charts and logs online via your preferred search engine.

For a quick boost of motivation look no further than modern media. Make a music playlist of songs that give you energy and/or fill you with determination. Watch a few health/workout videos online to see people who have successfully changed their lives through health and fitness to help you do the same.

Last but not least, find people that share your goals. Having support is a wonderful thing and will make it much easier to stay on track. Simply talking about our knowledge and progress on a regular basis will help us go that much further, not to mention that explaining something helps us to understand it even better. On the flip side, and this is important, spending time around influences (people, music, TV, movies) that reflect values that conflict with our goals can be very demotivating and slow our progress a great deal. Have you ever found yourself wanting to grab a drink after watching a TV program where the characters are constantly indulging in alcohol... yeah me too. The kinds of information we take in could be considered part of our diets so we want to make sure we are exposing ourselves to things that help us, not hinder us.

-Summary

- Immersion is powerful but comes with a price.
- Recording your efforts helps you to see progress
- Use energetic music and fitness videos for an extra boost
- Spend time with people who have similar goals to keep motivation high

Diet

———

Our diet consists of the fuel and nutrients we consume and will be an important angle to consider. Now, everyone is different, some people can eat meat, cheese and potatoes every day and still maintain a slender physique while others will notice weight gain taking in half as much "soul food" as these naturally skinny individuals. To become a healthier version of ourselves it shouldn't be necessary to jump into any kind of extreme to see results. One thing we can do is keep a log of everything we eat over the course of at least a couple of weeks. Once you have a good list of foods that you typically eat, take a look at the nutritional content of those foods one by one and write that down as well (online searches are marvelous things simply type in: "nutrition facts for _____" in your favorite search engine and/or check nutrition labels).

Now that we have a list of vitamins, minerals, fat, carbs, sugars, protein, cholesterol, fiber and calories for our preferred foods we can replace one or two of the items on your list that have very similar nutritional values, with food items of higher quality. Outside of exercise we essentially want to keep protein levels more or less consistent, trade unhealthy saturated fats and trans fats for unsaturated fats and perhaps cut some calories and sugars while taking in very similar amounts of vitamins and minerals as we are eating these things for a reason. To give an example, replacing all the beef in our diets with chicken will be a step up while still allowing us to get our meaty fix. Trading out ice creams, candy and soda pop with fruit will retain much of the sugar that we ingest but now we've added more vitamins and nutrients (I'm not joking when I say that fruit is nature's candy). Start as small as you want and work your way up to a fairly healthy diet that you'll be able to stick with as even small changes will produce results over time.

So you may be wondering how much to eat in a typical day. Well, it depends on what you typically do on a day to day basis, forget all that 2,000 calories per day nonsense as we are all spending energy differently in different amounts and furthermore eat more or less depending on the amount of muscle we have. Muscles require a lot of energy to be maintained by the body so by simply cultivating more muscle we can eat more often and keep our fat levels down.

I've noticed over the years that many women seem to be afraid of gaining too much muscle and then point out that guys are lucky that they seem to not gain body fat as easily. I assure the ladies out there that a little muscle goes a long way and you can still look great, it's worth it.

As for the frequency of our meals I would say to just experiment with it and find what seems to work best for you. We have the 3 meals a day paradigm that can be used as a base, and then as we add more meals, be sure to cut back on calories in each one and make sure it's well balanced no matter the size, think: (vegetables, source of protein, carbs, good fat, vitamins and minerals). Eating smaller meals more often can help keep the metabolism fired up as long as it's the same amount of food you would eat regularly just spread out. I tend to eat around 4-5 meals a day and that works well for me. If you are anything like my family you may not be so keen on vegetables and to that I say make green smoothies. Your smoothies should be based around a few vegetables and then have just enough fruit to strike a slightly sweet flavor or neutral if you wanted it to be on the more healthy side. I have also found that hot peppers are an interesting way to add more of an experience to your smoothies and has the added bonus of becoming a source of amusement to the people you would have try your concoction (PLEASE make sure they aren't allergic first).

On to some specifics on the various forms of nutrition in order of how they appear on the "Nutrition Facts" label on food and drinks:

-Calories:

To put it simply, calories are the amount of energy a food item contains. We essentially want to consume the amount of energy we wish to spend or else we store the excess as fat. Our Caloric needs change with our level of activity and further increase when we are breaking down and rebuilding muscle through exercise. Fats, carbohydrates and protein are the elements of food that contain calories and in some "Nutrition Facts" labels it will actually have the caloric value of each in this format:

Calories per gram:

Fat 9 • Carbohydrate 4 • Protein 4

Fat: As you can see above, fat is a dense source of energy so while eating fat doesn't necessarily cause us to gain more body fat, it can make it easier to consume more calories than we are going to spend.

Some vitamins are fat soluble, which means they require fat in order for our bodies to use them and shows the value of fat in our diets. There are "good" fats (unsaturated) and "bad" fats (saturated, Trans), reducing the amount of Trans and saturated fats is important because they can raise cholesterol levels.

Cholesterol is a type of fat in the blood and is necessary for some organ functions but only in small amounts.

Carbohydrates: Carbs are the body's go-to source of energy. They are used up first before we start tapping fats and proteins for energy. There are simple carbs (think sugars and white bread/ rice) and complex carbs (whole grains) and the difference between them is how quickly they are used with complex carbs being more slowly processed. **Fiber** is a type of carbohydrate but instead of being turned into energy, it is not broken down and aids in digestive health. Anyone who has been constipated or had hemorrhoids knows the value of fiber in the diet.

Protein: In order to rebuild muscles after exercise the body requires protein. Protein is also one of the elements responsible for helping us to feel full after eating. While protein is essential to building muscle, consuming large amounts of protein won't allow the muscle to grow beyond the amount of exercise you put into it so don't go thinking you can knock back several protein shakes and see massive gains.

-Sodium:

Sodium is most commonly consumed as table salt. It works with nerves, muscles and helps balance the fluids in our bodies. We over consume sodium mainly through processed foods as it is a preservative. Watch out for foods labeled as low fat and low sugar as they will often contain extra sodium for taste.

-Essential Vitamins and Minerals and what they are good for:

Vitamin A: Eyes

B Vitamins: Energy, immune system

Vitamin C: Skin, antioxidant

Vitamin D: Bones, mood (sunlight provides vitamin D)

Vitamin E: Skin, hair, nails

Vitamin K: Blood clotting

Calcium: Bones, Teeth

Iron: Muscle, blood

Zinc: Immune system, growth

Chromium: Energy

Last we have the matter of hydration. We are mostly made of water, so drinking lots of water is going to help us in every way imaginable (seriously, drink water). Last time I checked, the general recommendation for water consumption was 8, 8oz glasses of water a day which is a half-gallon a day. We are all different so we can use that as a base, if you aren't drinking a half gallon a day then start with that. Another point to consider is water weight or how much water our body retains at any given time (this can make us look kind of puffy). Our body holds onto more water depending on how little water we take in, as to preserve what it can while it has it. The more water you drink, the less inclined we are to indulge in sugary beverages like soda, which are pointless calories. So, drinking more water, more often will actually cause the body to let go of excess water weight, helping us to lose weight and have a more "cut" physique.

-Summary-

- Write down what you eat over the course of 2 weeks or so and research their nutritional content. Replace foods you eat with healthier alternatives.
- Eating 4+ small, balanced meals will help keep the metabolism running at a faster pace as opposed to the 3 meals a day paradigm.
- Fruit has sugar
- If you aren't a huge fan of vegetables, make green smoothies, just not too sweet or else you're defeating the purpose.

- Unsaturated fats are good in controlled amounts
- Cholesterol is useful in very small amounts
- Carbs are quick use energy, use it before it's stored away as fat
- Fiber helps your digestive system move smoothly
- Protein is useful but only consume as much protein as your body will use
- Processed foods have too much sodium
- Drink at least 8, 8oz glasses of water a day (half gallon)
- Drinking water helps us lose weight

Supplements

———

Multivitamins, protein powders, fat loss pills, fish oil... today's market is flooded with supplements claiming to offer enhanced health in a bottle. Humanity has existed on this planet for quite some time without the need for concentrated chemicals to achieve health and wellness so why are we bombarded with so many of them now? On one hand, the increased demand for food has led to the gradual decline in the nutritional content of mass produced food stuffs, leaving a nutritional void that could be filled by eating larger quantities of this food or through nutrition supplements like multivitamins. On the other hand, while it will take some effort, it's entirely possible to get all the nutrients you need by buying higher quality foods (at a higher price tag) or by starting a garden.

As far as supplements go, if you want to go that route, it should only be necessary to grab a multivitamin or a good quality greens supplement. While multivitamins will provide vitamins and minerals to help bridge the gap in your diet, it's important to consider what exactly is inside of these concentrated pills and how to use them most effectively. It is entirely possible to produce synthetic vitamins in a lab and while this is more cost effective, these synthetic variants aren't necessarily used by the body in the same way naturally occurring vitamins are. Also, when eating, we don't consume anywhere close to the magnitude of vitamins and minerals present in multivitamins which leaves us to wonder if the body is even able to process a whole multivitamin or if it just flushes the majority of it back out. To maximize the effectiveness of multivitamins, find one that is derived from natural ingredients and preferably one that isn't very potent so you can split up the dosage and/or a half dose in the morning and the other in the evening. I encourage you to read up on these subjects and decide for yourself whether or not you want to take a multivitamin.

The other option for filling the nutritional void is an all-natural, greens supplement. Greens supplements, while they are dried and powdered, are composed of natural ingredients and super foods to enhance your diet. While these types of supplements won't completely make up for the nutritional deficiencies of a modern diet in the west, they are a convenient compromise to help us along, though, be sure to check out what kind of sweeteners are in them.

When it comes to other types of supplements, it's perhaps best to find a way to get the ingredients they contain from eating healthy foods instead. For example, say you would like to enhance your fat loss and feel tempted to grab one of those fat loss pills you've seen advertised on TV. One of the major components to most fat loss supplements are diuretics. Diuretics help the body to flush out water, helping us to lose weight (in water). Also, fat loss drugs usually include some kind of stimulant to help suppress appetite and give energy to make up for the reduced calorie consumption. Alternatives to the qualities of fat loss pills would be green tea, for extra energy as well as being a natural diuretic, increased water intake to further assist in losing water weight as well as helping us to feel more full and making sure to consume ample amounts of protein in each meal to curb appetite.

Another popular supplement in the world of fitness is protein powder. When you drink something, as opposed to eating solids, the nutrients are more quickly absorbed into the body. This provides a smaller window than solid matter for the substances to be effectively used by the body. By drinking our protein we also have the opportunity to take in much more protein than we would otherwise eat. It shouldn't be necessary to take protein powder if we are consuming ample amounts of protein with every meal but if you should decide to go down this road, consider how much it's really helping you and if it's worth the extra effort for the liver and kidneys to process (that goes for all supplements).

-Summary-

- Supplements can be useful as long as we know what's in them and are well informed on how they work.
- Whenever possible, try to get what you need from fresh, healthy foods

Strength Training

———

In this section I will be discussing various techniques to work out all of our various muscle groups. For many, all the different exercises can be intimidating and I'll admit there are quite a few to choose from and many gadgets and gizmos to help you do them. The only thing you really need to know for working on different muscles groups is that one side uses pushing movements while its opposite works with pulling movements. To work the biceps, we pull our hands towards our shoulder, to work the triceps we extend the arm. Abs crunch in, lower back straightens out from a crunched position and so on. The internet is very accessible at this point in history so I will not be including pictures of how to perform the exercises as videos on the techniques are extremely available and it will keep the cost of the book down. Pick one exercise for each muscle group that appeals to you or seems most appropriate to your skill level and after 3 weeks to a month, swap techniques for each muscle group. The reason that we want to avoid doing the same exercises for too long, even if we are hitting every muscle group, is that our bodies are HIGHLY adaptive, which is to say that anything we do over and over will become progressively easier and consequently require less energy to perform over time. This, while useful from a work perspective, poses a bit of a problem for using exercise to lose weight and challenge our muscles into growing bigger and stronger and/or leaner.

The frequency of your workouts depends on if your goals are to cut or gain weight. It will be sufficient to start with two days of exercise a week as a minimum, splitting up the exercises with 1-3 days in between for rest and recuperation. I find that it takes about 3 days for all soreness to leave me after starting up an exercise routine from a long break, but I am fairly youthful so take an additional day if you think you need it as we want you to install the habit more than anything. After you get used to exercising regularly you will notice that it takes less time to recover and you will come to even enjoy being sore (mmm endorphins). Rest days are an important part of the exercise process as that is the time that our body's consolidate and reinforce what you learning not to mention repairing itself.

The number of sets and repetitions that you are to perform on any exercise also depends on if you want to get lean and/or bigger. As a rule, less repetitions and a more challenging motion (Around 5-8 repetitions) will help to build bigger muscles and more repetitions (around 10-14 repetitions) at a lighter load will build leaner muscles. There is much debate on this topic, so again, find what works for you through trial and error. I highly recommend purchasing at least one pair of dumbbells between 10 and 25 pounds depending on your current level of strength as they will open the door to many more exercises. For the sake of simplicity, most of the exercises won't require equipment.

Lower Body

The legs are very powerful and used to increased activity so we are looking at higher reps, around 12-24 or so for applicable exercises. Your glutes are very strong muscles that help you support and perform all sorts of everyday movements.

Calf's

-Calf Raises:

Stand upright with your feet firmly planted on a flat, level surface, around shoulder width apart and slowly raise yourself into the tip toed position and then back down again to a flat footed position.

Variations: Grab something heavy and hold it against your body around the stomach like a large book, wear a backpack with something heavy in it, bowling ball or heavy box. The exercise can also be done with dumbbells or a barbell in hand.

Advanced: Perform the calf raise on one leg, keeping the motion slow, controlled and with good balance.

Thighs

-Forward Leg Raise:

Sit on the edge of a chair or bed with your legs at a 90 degree angle and feet resting flat on the ground. While seated, slowly straighten out one or both legs until fully extended and then in a controlled manner then back to the starting point.

Variations: Stand with your feet firmly planted, shoulder width apart and slowly raise one leg as high as your flexibility allows while remaining in a controlled manner keeping good balance.

Advanced: Wear leg weights or incorporate fitness bands

-Reverse Leg Raise:

Lay stomach down on a bed while supporting yourself with your forearms and have your legs extended, hanging off of the bed starting at the knees. Slowly curl your legs to a 90 degree angle at the knees and then lower them back out.

Variations: Add ankle weights if you have them.

-Body weight squat:

Stand in an upright position, feet firmly planted on a flat surface about shoulder width apart. Slowly lower the body at the knees until the legs are at a 90 degree angle while keeping your back straight and eyes forward and then return to standing position.

Variations: Same as calf raises.

Advanced: Same as calf raises and you could also perform a controlled hop to further extend the exercise; just be sure to land softly.

Glutes

-Plank Leg Raises:

Support yourself on the ground with your hands and knees in a four legged position. Extend one leg out behind you, raise and lower it while keeping the leg fully extended focusing on flexing the butt and lower back muscles then switch legs.

Advanced: Assume and hold a plank position while performing the leg raises.

-Body weight squat:

Stand in an upright position, feet firmly planted on a flat surface about shoulder width apart. Slowly lower the body at the knees until the legs are at a 90 degree angle while keeping your back straight and eyes forward and then return to standing position. Emphasize the Glutes, they are very powerful.

Variations: Same as calf raises.

Advanced: Same as calf raises and you could also perform a controlled hop to further extend the exercise; just be sure to land softly.

Mid Body

The abs, oblique's (love handle area) and lower back are very important muscles that help support us in everything we do. A weak core is a great way to invite injury into your life and lower back problems are very common these days.

Abs

-Crunches:

Lay down flat on the ground with your knees bent at roughly 90 degrees. The goal of the crunch is to strengthen the abdominal muscles, not to jerk ourselves up and down and we must be weary of straining the neck. In order to avoid some of the jerkiness from being new to the exercise you can place your fingertips around each hear and hold them there to avoid pulling on the neck. Focusing on the upper abs (roughly between the navel and lower ribs) slowly raise your torso up about 45 degrees until you can't go further and lower yourself back down.

Variations: After accustomed to the exercise try switching from slow controlled motions to doing them as fast as you can, avoid neck strain.

-Leg Crunch:

Lay down flat on the ground with your hands by the butt or lower back for support. Raise both legs together while fully extended to about 45 degrees and slowly lower them back down while focusing on the lower abdominals (Navel and below).

Variations: In the same position, cycle your legs in the air as if you were pedaling an imaginary bike. Try slowly scissoring your legs in the air for more variation.

-Side Crunch:

Lay down flat on one side with your top leg hovering around 35 degrees. While keeping your top arms elbow tucked into your side, pull your body up, sideways as far as it goes and lower back down focusing on the muscles to the side of your abs. This is a small kind of awkward movement but it works well so long as you stay focused on the muscles you are trying to work.

-Plank:

Drop down to the push up position but instead of supporting yourself on your hands, do so with your forearms. While keeping the back straight and level with the ground, hold the position for around 30 seconds and work on extending the time.

Advanced: While in plank, slowly with control, extend the right arm and left leg out then return to neutral plank and repeat with other arm and leg. This further works on our core strength and includes more shoulder, butt, leg and lower back.

Lower Back

-Standing Back Extension:

Stand up straight with legs shoulder width apart and arms crossed over the chest. Keeping your legs straight, slowly lower your torso 90 degrees at this hips and slowly return to upright position focusing on the lower back. For a lot of people nowadays the lower back is a sensitive area so be mindful of your movements and avoid jerking and fast motions.

Variations: Hold onto a decently sized book or another item with some weight at the chest. Be wary of advancing too quickly in weight to avoid injury.

-Plank Leg Raises:

Support yourself on the ground with your hands and knees in a four legged position. Extend one leg out behind you, raise and lower it while keeping the leg fully extended focusing on flexing the butt and lower back muscles then switch legs.

Advanced: Assume and hold a plank position while performing the leg raises.

Upper Body

Ah, the upper body, this is where we have all the so called glamour muscles such as the biceps, triceps, forearms, chest, back and shoulders. It's almost as though arm movements are more human in nature, perhaps this is why they are favored among many but in my humble opinion, huge arms and chest with ever shrinking muscular development as we descend down looks just plain silly; especially with the most exaggerated form of this imbalance commonly referred to as chicken leg syndrome. To help encourage you to spread your development evenly, in my experience, neglecting parts of ourselves in favor of others actually slows down overall gains, even in the area you're overemphasizing; and then of course it encourages injury. Balance balance balance.

Middle-Upper Back

-Rows:

Taking on too much too soon with this exercise can strain the lower back if in standing position so use good judgment. Grab an item of decent weight that can be gripped symmetrically between both hands such as a backpack loaded with books or a suitcase. Stand in an upright position and lower your torso at the hips about 90 degrees while holding the weighted item firmly in both hands with arms extended. While remaining bent over, slowly, with control, pull the weight to your body between the navel and ribs, flexing and focusing on the middle of the back and lower it back down.

Variations: Use differently weighted items to increase difficulty such as progressively heavier loads of laundry in a basket. Find a bed and rest one knee and hand on it while the other foot is on the ground and your other hand has the weight. Hold yourself steady and starting with your arm fully extended, hanging down, slowly pull the weight to the side of your body and back down.

Advanced: Do the standing or kneeling rows with dumbbells. Remember if using an item in each hand that they are to be brought to your sides, not above the navel.

-Chin ups:

The difference between a chin up and a pull up is in the grip. Chin ups have the palm facing away from you and pull ups have the palms inward. If you don't have access to a suitable bar or one of those door frame models, you can grab or buy a length of some kind of rope and toss it around a nice, thick tree branch. Stand up straight and grab the bar or rope at full arm extension and pull yourself up using your arms and back until your chin is over your hands.

Variations: If you cannot perform a chin up then grab a chair or something to give you extra height at a bar and then perform the movement from a squatting position using your legs as a support but only just enough to keep it difficult. The same technique can be used with the rope around a tree branch but if you have long enough rope then you can pull yourself up from a kneeling position.

Chest

-Dips:

Find a chair without arms, bench, or sturdy bed and stand in front of it facing away. Grab the edge of the surface with both hands, slightly behind your body and lower yourself using only your arms, chest and shoulders until your arms are bent 90 degrees and then raise yourself up by extending the arms and repeat while holding the tension.

-Bench press:

Find a bench or lay down on a flat surface. If you don't have dumbbells then you can use two, gallon jugs of a drink. Carefully extend your arms straight above your chest with the weights and then slowly lower them to your chest until your arms are about 90 degrees (or a little more if you are on a bench) and then back up focusing on the chest and arms. It is important to pay attention to your abs (core) for support and your upper back should be flexed to support the lowering motion while the chest moves the weights away from the body.

Variations: Rather than have your elbows come down perpendicularly to your torso, you can keep the elbows tucked in at your sides for the exercise.

-Push up:

While the push up tends to emphasize the chest and triceps, you will also be using the biceps for stability and control. If you cannot do a push up then use your knees instead of your feet for support which makes it roughly twice as easy and work up to a regular push up.

Variations: Place your hands closer together to perform a diamond push up; it will target the inner chest and triceps more. Placing your hands wider apart will work the outside of the chest more. **Decline Push up:** Perform the exercise with your feet resting on an elevated surface such as a step, bucket or chair. Decline push-ups target the upper chest and shoulders. **Incline push up:** Perform the exercise with your hands resting on an elevated surface like a step, bucket or chair. Incline push-ups work more on the lower chest.

Advanced: Perform weighted push-ups by wearing a backpack with some books in it. Keep in mind that you'll want the weight on the upper part of the back, directly above the arms so adjust the back pack accordingly and with books in a suitable place (stuff some shirts or towels to help prop up objects).

Biceps

-Bicep curls:

If you do not own dumbbells then you could use a bucket with some water in it, a briefcase with books in it, a large purse of suitable weight, an appropriate weighted tool box, a backpack or bag (maybe a grocery bag) with stuff in it or a gallon jug of some kind of drink. Standing upright with feet shoulder width apart, hold the weight down at your side with one arm, keep your palms facing out and moving only at the elbow, raise the object almost as far as your arm allows and then slowly lower back down. This exercise can be done with one or both arms at once as long as the weight is even in each hand.

Variations: Perform the curl with a neutral grip (palms facing the hips) to emphasize the other part of the bicep.

-Push up:

While the push up tends to emphasize the chest and triceps, you will also be using the biceps for stability and control. If you cannot do a push up then use your knees instead of your feet for support which makes it roughly twice as easy and work up to a regular push up.

Variations: Place your hands closer together to perform a diamond push up; it will target the inner chest and triceps more. Placing your hands wider apart will work the outside of the chest more.

Advanced: Perform weighted push-ups by wearing a backpack with some books in it. Keep in mind that you'll want the weight on the upper part of the back, directly above the arms so adjust the back pack accordingly and with books in a suitable place (stuff some shirts or towels to help prop up objects).

-Pull up:

See chin up but with your palms facing towards you.

Triceps

-Triceps Extension:

This exercise is like a reverse curl as you are extending the arm instead of curling it in. If you don't have a dumbbell try a gallon jug of some drink. Find a table or bed to lean on and bend over between 45-90 degrees with the elbow of the arm you are working tucked in at your side with the weight hanging down. Extend the arm, moving only at the elbow focusing on flexing the muscles opposite to the biceps.

-Dips:

Find a chair without arms, bench, or sturdy bed and stand in front of it facing away. Grab the edge of the surface with both hands, slightly behind your body and lower yourself using only your arms, chest and shoulders until your arms are 90 degrees and then raise yourself up by extending the arms and repeat while holding the tension.

-Push-up:

As you can see, push-ups are a formidable tool to exercising the upper body as well has building up core strength for stability.

-Overhead Triceps Extension:

This exercise will require a weighted object that you can comfortably hold above and behind your head with both hands. If you don't have a suitable dumbbell grab a large book, gallon jug, backpack, briefcase, purse and while standing up straight with feet shoulder width apart, raise the object over your head with arms full extended and then slowly lower it, bending the arms only at the elbows until the weight is behind your head and then extend your arms back over your head. Be sure you aren't going to hurt yourself from low ceilings and/or ceiling fans.

Forearms

While the forearms are used in most of the exercises it couldn't hurt to do a bit of training on them which will help strengthen the wrists and grip strength.

-Wrist curls:

If you don't have a small dumbbell, use a book. Sit in an arm chair and rest your arm with your elbow at the edge so your forearm and hands are hanging off. Take the weighted object and slowly move only your hands as far down as they go and up while focusing on the forearms.

Shoulders

Be mindful that the shoulders can be overworked if you are also performing many chest exercises. It would be a good idea to split up chest and shoulder days.

-Overhead Press:

This can be done while standing or sitting, the difference being that sitting will have you engage fewer muscles for support. If you don't have dumbbells you can use two, gallon jugs of liquid, carefully bring the weights above your head with arms fully extended and then lower the weights to the shoulders without actually resting them there and raise them back up.

-Push-ups:

Refer to previous sections

-Arm Raises:

Again, if you don't have dumbbells then gallon jugs with liquid work just fine, also books, and grocery bags with items and so on. Stand up straight with feet shoulder width apart, holding your weights in both hands at your sides. Slowly raise your arms up until you are in a T shape and then lower them back down focusing on the shoulder muscles.

Variations: This exercise can also be done by raising your arms out in front of you until level with your shoulders.

-Shrugs:

Grab two items of equal weight in each hand and while standing up straight, raise both of your shoulders up in the air while keeping the rest of your body still. This is a very simple exercise and easy too. It will work the muscles that rest between your shoulders and neck which also extend over the top of the back just under the neck.

-Summary-

- Pick out and write down one exercise for each muscle group that you would like to do. Keep in mind that some of the exercises: squats, jogging, cycling, push-ups and dips work several muscles groups at the same time and because of this you could use a couple of push up variations to serve as your chest, shoulder and triceps exercise which will cut down on workout time. Switch the exercises up every 3+ weeks.

- Many common household items can be used as adjustable weights, try out some of my examples and get creative just don't get upset if you put bricks in flimsy grocery bags and one breaks the bag and lands on your foot, that's on you.

- There are many ways to split up workouts, you can do all the exercises you've chosen in one day and then take 3 or so days off and do it again when you recover. You could work the front muscles of your body one day and then the next day work the back side. You could do your legs one day, torso the next and arms and shoulders last with a day or two of rest in between. Find what works well for you and your schedule.

- If you aren't challenged by your workout then you probably won't see much growth and development as our muscles grow in response to greater demand. Being sore the day after a workout is always a good sign but don't be surprised if you begin to recover much quicker.

Exercise List:

Lower Body:

Calf's:

- Calf Raises

Thighs:

- Forward Leg Raise
- Reverse Leg Raise
- Body Weight Squat ▲

Glute's:

- Plank Leg Raises
- Body Weight Squat ▲

Mid-Body:

Abs:

- Crunches
- Leg Crunch
- Side Crunch
- Plank

Lower Back:

- Standing Back extension
- Plank Leg Raises

Upper Body:

Middle-Upper Back:

- Rows
- Chin ups

Chest:

- Dips ♪
- Bench Press
- Push-ups ♥

Bicep's:

- Bicep Curls
- Push-ups ♥
- Pull ups

Triceps:

- Triceps Extensions
- Dips ♪
- Push-ups ♥
- Overhead Triceps extensions

Forearms:

- Wrist Curls

Shoulders:

- Overhead Press
- Push-ups ♥
- Arm Raises
- Shrugs

Cardio

———

In order for an exercise to be considered cardio, it must push the body into requiring extra oxygen through consistent effort and get the heart pumping faster (engage the cardiovascular system more). This sustained effort in exercising warms us up quickly and is great for strengthening and maintaining a healthy heart and lungs.

While strength training favors power and uses energy over time from tearing down and rebuilding muscle, cardio/endurance training taps into our carbohydrate supply rather quickly, making a good choice if you just want to burn through some extra calories. Long distance runners tend to be very lean and this is from the body taping into muscle and fat supplies after they have burned through their carbohydrates. The lean body of a long distance runner makes sense since they are training for endurance, therefore the body learns to use all of its fuel as efficiently as possible, holding onto only what's necessary to keep them going as extra weight would slow them down and cause more wear and tear on the legs and joints. You'll notice that sprinters don't necessarily have the leanness of the long distance runners, while they do engage the cardiovascular system, it's not to the extent that their body's burn through all excess energy and benefit from more muscular strength to hit top speed.

Jogging/running, jogging in place, power walking, jump roping, cycling or stationary cycling, jumping jacks, climbing stairs and swimming are the options for getting cardio into your routine. Depending on your current level of fitness, running might be tricky to get into right away so feel free to engage in power walking or another easier form of exercise. Stretching and going for a light walk before you start is a good idea to warm up the muscles and help avoid injury. The important thing here is to make it a habit and to progressively make it more difficult to maximize results. It's up to you whether you would like to go a more power oriented route with more effort and reduced time to help build and maintain muscle or endurance to lose weight and emphasize heart and lung health.

-Summary-

- Cardio requires sustained effort to work the heart and lungs

- Strength training helps maintain and build muscle while endurance training helps cut weight

- Before starting, warm up with stretching and a walk to help avoid injury

- Jogging/running, jogging in place, power walking, jump roping, cycling or stationary cycling, jumping jacks, climbing stairs and swimming are cardio exercises

Stretching

———

Stretching is very important to keep the body in working order. In this chapter I will give you some very basic exercises to get you going and I encourage you to expand your knowledge on the subject. Be mindful in your stretching and learn to enjoy the experience. Consider the differences in the bodies of the elderly and of children. Do we not get more stiff and restricted as we age? Stretching becomes even more important as we get older and given the focus on youthfulness these days, it is certainly something to add into our daily routine. Also try stretching at different times on days you work out, either before strength training, after strength training or in between exercises.

-Bends:

- **Calf:** Stand in front of a wall and step where the floor and wall meet so that your toes are on the wall and your heel is on the ground. Slowly apply light pressure so that you can feel it in your calf's.

- **Legs:** Stand up straight with feet shoulder width apart and slowly bend forward at the hips and try to touch your toes, stopping when it becomes painful. The trick to this exercise is bending at the hips as we tend to try to bend our back to feel like we can reach lower. It's important to enjoy the experience of our exercise and not just the end result or we can inadvertently slow our progress for the illusion of success.

- **Sides:** Stand up tall with your arms fully extended straight over your head. Slowly lean left until your right side begins to stretch and repeat with other side.

- Stand up tall and place your right elbow behind your head, grasping it with your left hand. Slowly lean to the left and repeat with opposite elbow and direction.

- **Wrists/Forearms:** Place your fingertips into the palm of your other hand and slowly apply light pressure feeling tension in the top of your forearm, pulling the hand back towards you and then in the opposite direction with both hands

-Twists:

- Sit down on the ground with your legs straight out in front of you. While maintaining the posture, place the right leg over the left, resting the right foot next to the left knee. Then, with arm extended, place your left elbow to the right of your right knee and hold this twisted position. Repeat with opposite arm and leg.

- Stand up straight with your arms out in a T shape. Twisting only at the hips, turn 90 degrees to your left and hold. Repeat with the right.

- While standing, wrap your left arm under your right and lightly grasp your right shoulder with your right arm fully extended. Rotate at the hips to your left until you feel your back stretching and repeat with other arm and direction.

-Summary-

- Stretch everyday

- Flexibility is a quality of youthfulness

- Go ahead a do all the exercises and research more into the subject, it goes quite deep.

Example Schedules

——

Next to applicable exercises will be an example of the number of sets and repetitions in this format: (SETS-REPS).

4 Rest Days:

Sun	Mon	Tues	Wed	Thurs	Fri	Sat
Rest	Lower-Mid Body: **Stretch** Walk 10min **Calf Raises (3-10)** Squats (3-10) **Crunches (3-10)** Leg Crunches (3-10) **Plank Leg Raises (3-10)**	Upper-Body: **Stretch** Rows (3-10) **Pushups (3-10)** Wrist Curls (3-10) **Shrugs (3-10)**	Rest	Cardio: **Walk 10min** Stationary Cycling 15min	Rest	Rest

Simple Spread:

Sun	Mon	Tues	Wed	Thurs	Fri	Sat
Rest	Lower Body: **Stretch** Walk 15min **Calf Raises (3-10)** F. Leg Raise (3-10) **Squats (3-10)**	Mid Body: **Stretch** Crunches (3-10) **Plank (3-1min)** Standing Back Extension (3-10)	Rest	Upper-Body: **Stretch** Rows (3-10) **Pushups (3-10)** Dips (3-10) **Wrist Curls (3-10)** Arm Raises (3-10)	Cardio: **Walk 10min** Stationary Cycling 15min	Rest

Spaced with Stretching Emphasis:

Sun	Mon	Tues	Wed	Thurs	Fri	Sat
Stretch	Lower Body: **Stretch** Cycling 15 min **Squat (4-15)**	Stretch	Mid Body: **Stretch** Plank (3-1min) **Side Crunch (3-20)**	Stretch	Upper-Body: **Stretch** Pushups (3-10) **Chin ups (3-10)** Wrist Curls (3-10) **Shrugs (3-20)**	Cardio: **Stretch** Walk 15 min **Jumping Jacks 5 min**

Cardio Emphasis:

Sun	Mon	Tues	Wed	Thurs	Fri	Sat
Stretch	Mid Body/Cardio:	Cardio:	Stretch	Lower body/Cardio:	Rest	Upper-Body/Cardio:
	Stretch	**Stretch**		**Stretch**		**Stretch**
	Walk 10 min	Walk 10 min		Squat (4-15)		Pushups (3-10)
	Cycling 20 mins	**Swimming 30 min**		**Leg Raises (3-10)**		**Dips (3-10)**
	Crunches (3-10)			Walk 10 min		Walk 10 min
	Side Crunches (2-20)			**Jogging in Place 5 min**		**Power Walk 25 min**
	Plank (3-1min)					
	Standing Back Extension					

Balanced Spread:

Sun	Mon	Tues	Wed	Thurs	Fri	Sat
Stretch	Upper-Body/Cardio: **Stretch** Walk 10 min **Push-ups (3-10)** Dips (3-10) **Stationary Cycling 20 mins**	Mid Body: **Stretch** Walk 10 min **Crunch (3-10)** Plank (3-1min) **Standing back Extensions (3-10)**	Arms/Cardio: **Stretch** Walk 10 min **Arm Raises (3-10)** Bicep Curls (3-10)	Lower Body: **Stretch** Squats (3-15) **Leg Extensions (3-10)** Reverse Leg Extensions (3-10)	Stretch	Cardio: **Stretch** 10 min Walk **Jump Rope 10 mins**

Bonus

———

Focus is an extremely powerful tool for exercising and just about anything else. Surely the act of doing an exercise requires enough focus by default, right? Nope. Think of it like this, while you can multitask and still get work done, doesn't the product of our effort become something much greater when we are completely focused and determined on what we have set out to do? For example, I can surf the web while watching TV but I honestly can't say that I remember the TV program or what I was doing online all that well compared to doing one at a time. So how do we add more focus into our exercise? For one thing, avoid distractions like TV while exercising (unless of course you are watching a workout program).

To enhance our efforts while exercising place all of your focus on the area of the body you are working; slow movements aid this end. While doing a bicep curl, feel the bicep growing tenser then relaxing throughout the motion. As you perform your push-ups, imagine the chest and arms filling with energy and giving you the strength to do an extra few reps. I've had great success in imagining the muscle I'm exercising underneath the skin, being fed energy and growing in power as it's required in the exercise. Completely immerse yourself in the exercise for maximum benefit.

Something that I have found to be especially potent for keeping extra weight off is implementing exercise at an appropriate time after eating, especially if what you ate was something very carb/sugar heavy. Simple carbohydrates such as non-whole grain pastas, breads and sugar are our body's quickest acting supply of energy. Fat is our body's way of storing excess energy so if we consume lots of quick-use energy and then don't use it within the time frame that it's available then it gets stored as fat. Therefore if we eat a big bowl of ice cream or a large pasta dinner we should engage in some sort of physical activity afterword to both take advantage of the extra quick access energy and to avoid storing it as fat. Timing for this is important and for me personally, I have had great success by hopping on an exercise bike around 40 minutes after eating a lot of carbs (I bought a stationary bike stand since I already owned a bike) but figure out what timing seems most appropriate for you. Now, I am not a very gassy person but I have noticed that if I exercise after loading up on carbs then I tend to burp a few minutes into my workout which indicates to me that I have started tapping into the energy of what I had eaten. Going for a walk, walking the dog, cleaning up a few rooms in the house at a good pace or some kind of strength training and stretching would be good routes to burn through the extra energy.

Try contemplating on how your body looks and feels and how these attributes help or hinder you from achieving your goals on a daily basis. Anything done repeatedly, over time, will yield skill and understanding and this goes for dieting and exercise too. If you continue to strive for a healthier lifestyle you will slowly begin to feel what the body needs to eat and what to do to enhance your health and that's when things get fun.